PEACEMARK SURGERY DIETARY

Complete Guide Unlocking The Secrets Of
Nutrition To Rapid Healing After Surgery
Success, Nourishing Meal Plans, Recipes, Tips
For Optimal Health Wellness

DR. ALLAN FREDA

Contents

INTRODUCTION 4

CHAPTER 1 10

THE BASICS OF PEACEMAKER SURGERY 12

CHAPTER 2 15

THE SCIENCE BEHIND DIETS FOR PEACEMAKER
SURGERY 15

CHAPTER 3 20

GETTING YOUR KITCHEN READY FOR SUCCESS
....20

CHAPTER 4 26

HOW WHOLE FOODS CAN HELP YOU FEEL
BETTER 26

CHAPTER 6 37

MAIN DISHES THAT SATISFY AND FEED 37

CHAPTER 7 40

SIDES AND SALADS THAT ENERGISE AND
REFRESH 40

CHAPTER 8 48

SWEET TREATS TO HELP YOU GET BETTER 48

CHAPTER 9 53

DRINKS THAT CAN HELP YOU HEAL AND STAY
HYDRATED 53

CHAPTER 10 60

HOW TO PLAN MEALS AND COOK IN BIG GRIPS 60

CHAPTER 11..66

DEALING WITH DIETARY PROBLEMS AND LIMITATIONS 66

CHAPTER 12..73

BEYOND THE PLATE: HOLISTIC APPROACHES TO HEALING...73

CONCLUSION 79

PeaceMark Surgery Dietary" focuses on the important part of nutrition after surgery, highlighting how important it is for healing and long-term health. It is a complete guide for people who have just been diagnosed and are going to have surgery. It contains a lot of useful information, such as healing recipes, carefully planned meals, and expert advice to help with the best recovery and s

INTRODUCTION

How to Read and Understand the Peacemaker Surgery Dietary Cookbook:

The road to recovery after peacemaker surgery can be difficult and important for patients. Diet plays a big part in this process, affecting healing and overall health. The Peacemaker Surgery Dietary Cookbook is a great resource to help people figure out how to eat properly after surgery. It has a lot of useful information, like healing recipes, m

A pacemaker is implanted during peacemaker surgery, which is a common way to treat irregular heart rhythms (arrhythmias). The surgery involves putting in a small electronic device called a pacemaker, which helps control the heart's electrical activity and keep the heartbeat normal. While the surgery itself is very important for treating heart problems, the time afterward is very important for making sure of a full recovery and minimizing complications.

It's very important to think about what you eat after surgery because nutrition is a big part of helping the body heal and improving your overall health.

The Peacemaker Surgery Dietary Cookbook understands how important customized nutrition is for recovery and gives people who are going through this life-changing journey useful advice.

Tips for Getting the Most Out of This Cookbook:

Using the Peacemaker Surgery Dietary Cookbook correctly is important for getting the best results in recovery after surgery.

This section explains the most important things people can do to get the most out of the cookbook, so they can make smart food choices that will help their healing.

1. Get to Know the Healing Recipes: The cookbook has a wide range of healing recipes carefully chosen to help with recovery after surgery. These recipes are carefully made to provide essential nutrients, speed up healing, and accommodate dietary restrictions that are common after peacemaker surgery. Take the time to look through the different recipes, paying close attention to the ingredients and nutritional profiles to make sure they fit your needs.

Plan Balanced Meals: It's important to plan your meals so that you can keep a healthy, well-balanced diet after surgery.

 The cookbook has meal plans that are designed to help with recovery and long-term wellness.

These plans tell you how much food to eat, how to combine foods, and when to eat them. Stick to these meal plans to make sure you're getting all the nutrients you need while also healing and feeling healthy.

3. Include Expert Tips: The Peacemaker Surgery Dietary Cookbook has more than just recipes and meal plans. It also has expert tips and insights from cardiac care and nutrition experts. These tips cover a wide range of topics related to nutrition after surgery, such as dietary guidelines, staying hydrated, taking supplements, and ways to deal with common problems like changes in appetite or dietary restrictions.

4. Make it Fit Your Needs: The cookbook has a lot of helpful information and ideas, but it's important to make sure that its suggestions fit your wants and needs.

Talk to your doctor or a registered dietitian to create a personalized nutrition plan that takes into account things like your medical history, dietary restrictions, food allergies, and lifestyle choices. Then, use the cookbook as a base to build a diet plan that works for you.

5. Be Consistent and Patient: For the best results in recovery after surgery, you need to be consistent, patient, and committed to living a healthy life.

Have a positive attitude about the healing journey, knowing that progress may take time and persistence. Commit to following the dietary suggestions in the cookbook, and believe in the healing power of eating healthy foods.

Finally, the Peacemaker Surgery Dietary Cookbook is a complete guide to the best nutrition after surgery. It has a lot of helpful information, like healing recipes, meal plans, and expert tips that are designed to help with recovery and long-term health.

People who are having peacemaker surgery can take charge of their recovery by using the information and strategies in this cookbook and being proactive about their nutrition.

Disclaimer

The information in this book is for informational purposes only and should not replace professional medical advice, diagnosis, or treatment. Always consult your physician or a qualified health provider regarding any medical concerns. Do not disregard professional medical advice or delay seeking it based on information in this book.

The author does not endorse or have affiliations with any mentioned entities. References are for informational purposes only.

Consult your healthcare provider before making dietary or lifestyle changes, especially during recovery from surgery, as individual needs vary.

Results may vary, and the information provided is not guaranteed to produce specific outcomes.

By reading this book, you acknowledge and agree to consult your healthcare provider before implementing any information herein.

For further guidance, consult your healthcare provider or reputable medical websites for reliable information on surgery recovery diets.

CHAPTER 1
THE BASICS OF PEACEMAKER SURGERY

A common medical procedure called pacemaker surgery involves putting a small electronic device called a pacemaker into the chest to help control irregular heartbeats. The pacemaker sends electrical impulses to the heart to make it beat at a normal rate, which makes sure that blood flows properly throughout the body. People who have conditions like bradycardia (slow heart rate) or arrhythmias (irregular heart rhythms) that can't be treated with medicine are often told to have this surgery.

What is surgery for a pacemaker?

The goal of pacemaker surgery, which is also called implantation of a cardiac pacemaker, is to put a small electronic device under the skin near the collarbone.

This device, called a pacemaker, helps keep the heartbeat normal by sending electrical impulses to the heart muscles. The pacemaker is made up of a pulse generator and leads, which are thin, insulated wires that connect the generator to the heart.

How diet is an important part of getting better

A healthy diet is very important for getting better after pacemaker surgery. It can help the body heal, lower the risk of complications, and improve overall heart health. After surgery, the body needs the right nutrients to repair tissues, boost the immune system, and keep energy levels up. Some food choices can also help with conditions that may have caused the need for the surgery in the first place, like hype.

How the Foods You Choose Can Affect Your Healing

What you eat can have a big effect on how quickly you heal after pacemaker surgery. A diet high in essential nutrients like vitamins, minerals, antioxidants, and protein can help repair tissues and lower inflammation.

Fresh fruits and vegetables, whole grains, lean proteins, and healthy fats are all important parts of a healing-oriented diet. These foods give the body the building blocks it needs for cell regeneration, immune function, and heart health.

CHAPTER 2

THE SCIENCE BEHIND DIETS FOR PEACEMAKER SURGERY

Peacemaker surgery, also called pacemaker surgery, is a very important medical procedure that controls irregular heart rhythms. Understanding the science behind what you need to eat after surgery is important for a speedy recovery and good long-term health. This section goes into detail about the complicated physiology of healing, lists the foods you need after surgery, and stresses how important balanced nutrition is in the recovery process.

Looking into the Physiology of Healing

After surgery, the body goes through a complicated process to heal. Right away, it starts the inflammatory response to protect itself from infection and start repairing the tissue.

This is followed by the proliferative phase, where new tissue is made, and finally, the remodeling phase, where the healed tissue gets stronger and more flexible. Each of these phases needs different nutrients to help it work.

In peacemaker surgery, the heart is put under a lot of stress and trauma, so it needs the right nutrients to help it heal and grow back. Nutrients like protein, vitamins, minerals, and antioxidants are very important at different stages of healing.

For example, protein is needed to repair tissues and build muscles, and vitamins and minerals help enzymes do their job, which is very important for wound healing.

Needs for Nutrition After Surgery

Following surgery for a pacemaker involves a lot of different nutritional needs. These needs include helping the wound heal and maintaining good heart health. Getting enough protein is very important because it helps repair tissues and keeps muscles from losing mass, which is especially important for people having heart procedures. Lean meats, fish, eggs, dairy products, legumes, and nuts are all good sources of protein.

Also, getting enough micronutrients like vitamin C, vitamin E, zinc, and selenium is important for their roles in antioxidant defense and collagen synthesis. These nutrients help fight oxidative stress, lower inflammation, and speed up tissue regeneration. Omega-3 fatty acids, which can be found in fatty fish, flaxseeds, and walnuts, may also help with heart health, making them great foods to eat after surgery.

Complex carbohydrates from whole grains, fruits, and vegetables give you long-lasting energy and fiber for regular bowel movements, which can be affected by anesthesia and painkillers after surgery. Staying hydrated is also important to avoid problems like constipation, urinary tract infections, and electrolyte imbalances, so patients should drink a lot of fluids, preferably water, herbal teas, and sports drinks.

Why balanced nutrition is important for recovery

A well-balanced, nutrient-dense diet is an important part of healing from peacemaker surgery because it improves overall health and the body's ability to heal and adapt. Poor nutrition can weaken the immune system, slow down wound healing, and raise cardiovascular risk factors, all of which slow down the healing process. This is why healthcare professionals stress the importance of eating in ways that prioritize whole, minimally processed foods.

Maintaining a healthy weight and improving cardiovascular health through diet can also help stop complications and lower the risk of future cardiac events. Eating a plant-based diet high in fruits, vegetables, whole grains, and healthy fats can have a positive effect on lipid profiles, blood pressure, and glucose control, making the cardiovascular system less stressed and promoting long-term we

the research behind peacemaker surgery diets shows how important nutrition is for healing, heart health, and long-term health. By understanding how the body heals, meeting specific nutritional needs after surgery, and stressing the importance of balanced nutrition for recovery, healthcare professionals can improve patient outcomes and quality of life for people who are going through surgery.

CHAPTER 3

GETTING YOUR KITCHEN READY FOR SUCCESS

When you start a new diet after surgery, getting your kitchen ready is very important.

A well-equipped kitchen that is stocked with healing ingredients and organized for efficiency sets the stage for the best recovery and long-term health. In this section, we'll talk about the most important tools and equipment, how to stock your pantry with healing ingredients, and how to plan and organize meals for efficiency.

Important Tools and Equipment

When you're on a diet after surgery, buying the right tools and equipment can speed up the process and make meal preparation easier and faster.

1. Blender or food processor: You can't make smoothies, soups, or purees without these tools,

which are often suggested in the early stages of healing.

2. Sharp knives and a cutting board: Cutting fruits, veggies, and other foods safely and accurately is easier with a good set of knives and a hard-cutting board.

3. Steamer Basket: This is the best way to cook veggies while keeping their natural flavors and nutrients.

4. A slow cooker or an instant pot: These are great for making healthy meals with little work since you can just set them and forget about them.

5. Measuring cups and spoons: It's important to measure items correctly so you can follow recipes and make sure you're serving the right amount.

6. Good cookware: Buy pots, pans, and baking sheets that spread heat evenly to keep food from burning or cooking unevenly.

By getting these important tools for the kitchen, you'll be ready to make meals after surgery quickly and easily.

Stocking Your Kitchen with Good for You Foods

For a healthy diet after surgery, it's important to keep your pantry filled with healing foods. Here are some staples to include:

1. Whole Grains: Choose foods that are high in nutrients, like quinoa, brown rice, oats, and whole wheat pasta. These foods will give you long-lasting energy and the minerals you need to heal.

2. Lean Proteins: To help your muscles heal and you recover overall, eat foods like chicken breast, turkey, fish, tofu, and beans that are high in lean protein.

Healthy Fats: To help you feel full and absorb nutrients better, eat foods like avocados, nuts, seeds, and olive oil that are high in healthy fats.

4. Fresh Fruits and veggies: Stock your pantry and fridge with a wide range of colorful fruits and veggies that are high in antioxidants, vitamins, and minerals to help your immune system work better and speed up the healing process.

5. Low-Sodium Broths and Stocks: These flexible foods can be used as the base for healthy soups and stews. They add water and important nutrients without adding too much sodium.

6. Herbs and spices: Garlic, ginger, turmeric, basil, and parsley are some herbs and spices that can make your food taste better and also help reduce inflammation.

7. Healthy Snacks: To keep you from getting too hungry between meals, keep healthy snacks like Greek yogurt, hummus, fresh fruit, nuts, and whole-grain bread on hand.

Stocking your pantry with these healing foods will give you the tools you need to make healthy meals that will help you recover and stay healthy in the long run.

Making meal plans and organizing them to save time

Keeping up with a diet after surgery requires careful planning and organization of meals. Here are some tips to help you plan and organize your meals better:

1. Make a weekly meal plan. At the start of each week, take some time to plan out your meals, taking into account any dietary restrictions, nutritional needs, and personal tastes. This will help you stay on track and avoid making hasty decisions at the last minute that could lead to unhealthy choices.

2. Prepare the ingredients ahead of time: Wash, chop, and measure out ingredients once a week to make food preparation easier and faster. Put the prepared ingredients in airtight containers and keep them in the fridge for easy access all week.

3. Batch cook: Make big batches of basic foods like soups, grains, and proteins that can be divided up and kept for quick and easy meals during the week. This saves time and makes sure you always have healthy options on hand.

4. Use Leftovers: Don't throw away leftovers; use them in other meals or make new dishes with them to keep your diet interesting and reduce food waste.

Keep an open mind: Having a meal plan is helpful, but you should be able to change your mind if your schedule or dietary needs change. Always have a range of ingredients on hand that can be used in different recipes.

When you use these planning and organizing tips, making meals will go more quickly and easily. This will make it easier to follow your post-surgery diet plan and live a healthy life for long-term health.

CHAPTER 4
HOW WHOLE FOODS CAN HELP YOU FEEL BETTER

When it comes to recovering from surgery, nutrition is very important. A well-balanced diet is key to speeding up the healing process, building muscle, and improving overall health. Whole foods, in particular, are very important to include in your post-surgery diet. These naturally occurring, nutrient-dense foods are full of vitamins, minerals, antioxidants, and phytonutrients that help the body heal.

Fresh fruits and vegetables should be used.

Fresh fruits and vegetables serve as cornerstones of a post-surgery diet, delivering an array of vital nutrients to aid in the healing process. Rich in vitamins, such as vitamin C and vitamin E, as well as minerals like zinc and magnesium, fruits and vegetables bolster the immune system, reduce inflammation, and facilitate tissue repair. Additionally, they are abundant sources of dietary fiber, which aids in digestion, prevents constipation—a common postoperative issue—and promotes gut health. Incorporating a diverse array of colorful fruits and vegetables ensures a broad spectrum of nutrients essential for optimal recovery.

Leafy greens like spinach and kale offer an abundance of vitamins and minerals, while vibrant berries provide antioxidants that combat oxidative stress and support cellular health.

Furthermore, cruciferous vegetables such as broccoli and Brussels sprouts boast anti-inflammatory properties, aiding in the reduction of swelling and discomfort post-surgery.

By incorporating ample servings of fresh fruits and vegetables into post-surgery meals and snacks, individuals can nourish their bodies and expedite the healing process.

Lean proteins are important for recovery.

Protein plays a pivotal role in post-surgery recovery, serving as the building blocks for tissue repair and regeneration. Lean proteins, in particular, offer an optimal source of high-quality protein without the excess saturated fat found in many animal-based products.

Incorporating lean proteins into the post-surgery diet provides essential amino acids necessary for wound healing and muscle restoration. Sources such as poultry, fish, tofu, legumes, and low-fat dairy products offer an array of options to meet protein needs while promoting satiety and sustaining energy levels.

Additionally, incorporating omega-3 fatty acids from fatty fish like salmon and trout can further enhance the anti-inflammatory properties of the diet, supporting the body's healing process.

Including protein-rich foods at each meal and snack not only aids in recovery but also helps prevent muscle loss—a common concern during periods of immobility post-surgery. By prioritizing lean proteins in the post-surgery diet, individuals can support optimal healing and regain strength more efficiently.

Whole grains and legumes that are good for you

Whole grains and legumes serve as valuable additions to the post-surgery diet, offering a multitude of health benefits to aid in recovery and long-term wellness.

Rich in complex carbohydrates, fiber, vitamins, and minerals, whole grains provide sustained energy and promote digestive health. Options such as brown rice, quinoa, oats, and whole wheat pasta offer nutrient-dense alternatives to refined grains, which lack the fiber and essential nutrients found in their whole counterparts.

Moreover, legumes such as beans, lentils, and chickpeas deliver a hearty dose of plant-based protein, fiber, and micronutrients, making them valuable components of a post-surgery meal plan. These nutrient-rich foods contribute to feelings of fullness, stabilize blood sugar levels, and support cardiovascular health—a critical aspect of overall wellness, especially during the recovery period. Incorporating beneficial whole grains and legumes into post-surgery recipes and meal plans not only enhances nutritional intake but also promotes long-term health and well-being.

whole foods are very important for speeding up recovery after surgery and promoting long-term health. By focusing on fresh fruits and vegetables, lean proteins, and healthy whole grains and legumes in the post-surgery diet, people can give their bodies the nutrients they need for healing, repair, and vitality. Eating a variety of whole foods not only speeds up recovery but also sets the stage for long-term health.

How to Make Soups That Taste Great and Are Full
of Good Things for You

As an important part of peacemaker surgery diets, soups:

People who are having peacemaker surgery should eat a lot of soups because they are easy to make and full of nutrients that help the body heal. Soups are perfect for this because they are comforting and can be changed to fit each person's diet.

Soups are great for people who have recently had surgery because they are easy to change to fit different dietary needs or preferences. When people are recovering from peacemaker surgery, it is important to focus on eating nutrient-dense foods that help the body heal and stay healthy. For example, choosing lean proteins, whole grains, and a variety of vegetables can help their bodies heal and stay healthy.

Also, soups naturally contain a lot of water, which is especially important during the recovery period after surgery. Staying hydrated is important for helping the body heal and avoiding problems like dehydration, which can slow down the recovery process. Soups are a great way to stay hydrated, especially when made with broth or stock-based liquids, which can help patients keep their fluid levels at the right level during the recovery process.

Soups are not only good for you, but they are also easy to make in large amounts, which makes them a great choice for people who may not have much energy or mobility after surgery. Making a batch of soup ahead of time means that patients can have healthy meals ready to go without having to do a lot of planning or cooking. This can be especially helpful in the early stages of recovery when energy levels may be low, and the

Broth and stock recipes that are good for you:

People who are recovering from peacemaker surgery should make sure that the soups they eat are made with ingredients that are both healthy and easy on the digestive system. Broths and stocks are the base of many soup recipes and are full of nutrients like vitamins, minerals, and amino acids that help the body heal.

For post-surgery diets, homemade broths and stocks are better because you can control more of the ingredients and make them fit your specific needs and tastes. To make a healthy broth or stock, start with good ingredients like bones, vegetables, and herbs and simmer them over low heat to get the most flavor and nutrients out of them. Bone broths are especially popular because they contain a lot of collagen, which can help with recovery.

When choosing ingredients for homemade broths and stocks, choose nutrient-dense foods like chicken, beef, or fish bones, as well a variety of vegetables and herbs. Carrots, celery, onions, and garlic are common additions that give homemade broths and stocks more flavor and nutritional value. You could also add herbs and spices like parsley, thyme, and bay leaves to improve the flavor and provide extra health benefits.

For people who don't have the time or energy to make their broths and stocks from scratch, store-bought alternatives can also be good. Look for low-sodium options made from natural ingredients, and add extra vegetables or protein sources to make them more nutritious. Using healthy broths and stocks in soup recipes after surgery is a great way to give your body the nutrients it needs.

Different kinds of creative soup for all tastes:

Traditional chicken noodle soup may be a classic choice for recovering from surgery, but there are a lot of creative variations that can suit a wide range of tastes and dietary needs. For example, people who may be on a restricted diet during their recovery may find that experimenting with different flavor combinations and ingredients keeps meals interesting and fun.

For example, you could add seasonal vegetables like squash, sweet potatoes, or leafy greens to soups to make them look better, taste better, and be healthier.

Roasting vegetables before adding them to soups can bring out their natural sweetness and depth of flavor, making a hearty dish that is both healthy and tasty.

Along with vegetables, you might want to add protein sources like beans, lentils, or tofu to soups to make them filling and healthy. These plant-based protein options are great for people who are on a vegetarian or vegan diet while they are recovering, and they can help with muscle repair and healing overall.

Also, trying out different herbs, spices, and seasonings can help make soups taste better without using too much salt or fat. For example, fresh herbs like basil, cilantro, and mint can make soups taste brighter and fresher, while spices like cumin, turmeric, and ginger can make them taste deeper and more complex.

Overall, the best way to make creative soup variations is to use high-quality ingredients, try out different flavor combinations, and include a variety of nutrient-dense foods. By being open to new ideas and trying new things, people who are recovering from peacemaker surgery can enjoy a wide range of tasty and healthy soups that help them heal and promote their long-term health.

CHAPTER 6

MAIN DISHES THAT SATISFY AND FEED

It's important to eat nutrient-dense foods after surgery to help your body heal and recover as quickly as possible. Main dishes that are both satisfying and healthy are very important to post-surgery diet plans because they provide the nutrients, energy, and satisfaction that your body needs to heal and be healthy overall. Whether you're a meat-lover, a vegetarian, or a vegan, eating a variety of protein-packed and healthy meals can a

Protein-rich meals to help you recover

Because proteins are the building blocks of tissues, muscles, and cells, they are very important for recovery after surgery. Eating protein-rich main dishes is a great way to rebuild and repair the body's tissues, which helps with healing and strength. Lean sources of protein like chicken, fish, turkey, eggs, tofu, and legumes can give you the amino acids you need for muscle regeneration and tissue repair.

Vegetarian and vegan options that are good for you

Plenty of healthy options for vegetarians and vegans to meet their protein needs and help their recovery after surgery. Plant-based proteins like chickpeas, lentils, quinoa, tofu, tempeh, nuts, and seeds are great sources of protein, fiber, vitamins, and minerals. Adding these to main dishes like lentil soup, tofu stir-fry, chickpea curry, or quinoa salad with roasted vegetables can help your body recover.

How to Balance Macronutrients for Best Healing

In addition to protein, it's important to balance macronutrients like fats and carbohydrates for the best healing and recovery after surgery. Carbohydrates give the body energy, which is important for supporting cellular functions and promoting healing.

Choose complex carbohydrates like whole grains, fruits, vegetables, and legumes to get long-lasting energy and important nutrients.

To sum up, main dishes that are filling and healthy are important parts of a post-surgery diet because they provide the nutrients and energy that are needed for healing and overall health. Whether you like protein-packed meals, vegetarian or vegan options, or a mix of the two, eating a variety of healthy foods with balanced macronutrients can help you recover quickly and stay healthy in the long term.

CHAPTER 7
SIDES AND SALADS THAT ENERGISE AND REFRESH

When it comes to what to eat after surgery, it's impossible to overstate how important it is to include energizing and refreshing sides and salads. These foods are essential for supporting the healing process and making sure that you recover as quickly as possible. Sides and salads have many benefits, such as providing essential nutrients, aiding digestion, promoting hydration, and improving overall health. In this detailed guide, we'll talk about the importance of i

How to Add Colourful Salads to Your Diet:

Salads constitute an integral component of a post-surgery diet due to their abundant nutrient content and hydrating properties. When preparing salads, focus on incorporating a diverse range of colorful vegetables, leafy greens, fruits, nuts, seeds, and lean proteins to maximize nutritional value. Incorporating a variety of ingredients ensures that you receive a wide spectrum of vitamins, minerals, antioxidants, and phytonutrients essential for tissue repair, immune function, and overall health. Opt for leafy greens such as spinach, kale, arugula, and romaine lettuce as the base of your salad, as they are rich in vitamins A, C, and K, and various minerals. Additionally, includes colorful vegetables like bell peppers, carrots, tomatoes, cucumbers, and beets to add flavor, texture, and a plethora of essential nutrients. Adding fruits such as berries, apples, oranges, and pomegranates can impart natural sweetness and provide an extra dose of vitamins and antioxidants. Furthermore, incorporating protein sources like grilled chicken, tofu, chickpeas, or quinoa enhances satiety and supports muscle repair and recovery. To elevate the nutritional profile of your salad, sprinkle it with heart-healthy fats from sources like avocado slices, nuts, seeds, or a drizzle of extra virgin olive oil. Experiment with various homemade dressings made from olive oil, lemon juice, vinegar, herbs, and spices to add flavor without compromising healthfulness. By incorporating vibrant salads into your post-surgery diet, you can nourish your body with essential nutrients, promote hydration, support healing, and enhance overall well-being.

Side dishes that are high in nutrients to help with healing:

In addition to salads, incorporating nutrient-dense side dishes into your post-surgery diet is crucial for supporting healing and optimizing recovery. Side dishes offer an excellent opportunity to pack a nutritional punch and ensure that your meals are well-rounded and balanced. When selecting side dishes, prioritize whole, unprocessed foods rich in vitamins, minerals, fiber, and antioxidants to promote healing and enhance overall health.

Opt for complex carbohydrates such as sweet potatoes, quinoa, brown rice, whole grain pasta, and legumes to provide sustained energy levels and support tissue repair.

These foods are rich in fiber, which aids digestion, regulates blood sugar levels, and promotes satiety. Additionally, includes a variety of colorful vegetables, steamed, roasted, or sautéed, to provide a wide array of vitamins, minerals, and phytonutrients essential for cellular repair and immune function.

Leafy greens like spinach, kale, and Swiss chard are particularly beneficial due to their high vitamin and mineral content. Incorporating lean proteins such as grilled fish, turkey, chicken, tofu, or beans into your side dishes is essential for supporting muscle repair, maintaining lean body mass, and promoting satiety.

Furthermore, incorporating healthy fats from sources like avocado, nuts, seeds, and olive oil enhances nutrient absorption and provides anti-inflammatory benefits.

Experiment with herbs, spices, and homemade sauces to add flavor and variety to your side dishes without relying on excessive salt or unhealthy additives. By incorporating nutrient-dense side dishes into your post-surgery diet, you can provide your body with the essential nutrients it needs to support healing, boost immunity, and optimize overall wellness.

How to Make Meals with Balanced Sides:

Making sure your post-surgery food meets your nutritional needs and helps you heal and recover as quickly as possible is key. Here are some tips to help you make well-rounded meals that are good for your health:

1. Make variety a priority. In your meals, try to include a variety of foods from all food groups, such as fruits, veggies, whole grains, lean proteins, and healthy fats. Variety makes sure that you get all the nutrients you need to heal and recover.

2. Portion Control: Watch your portions to avoid eating too much and feel full faster. Use smaller plates and bowls to help you keep track of your portions and stay away from too many calories.

3. Balance Macronutrients: Make sure your meals have the right amount of carbs, proteins, and fats to keep you full, help your muscles heal, and improve the absorption of nutrients. Eating a variety of macronutrients at each meal also makes you feel fuller and better overall.

4. Add color: Eat a range of colorful fruits and vegetables to get a lot of vitamins, minerals, and antioxidants that your body needs to heal and recover. Aim to fill half of your plate with fruits and vegetables to get the most nutrition and improve your health.

5. Mindful Eating: Pay attention to your body's signals of hunger and fullness, chew your food well, and enjoy every bite.

Eating carefully can help you avoid overeating, improve digestion, and make the whole dining experience better.

6. Staying hydrated: Drink a lot of water throughout the day to stay properly hydrated. Staying hydrated is important for digestion, keeping your body temperature in check, flushing out toxins, and supporting your general health and well-being.

7. Pay Attention to Your Body: Pay attention to what your body is telling you and change your diet based on what it tells you. If certain foods or ingredients make you feel bad or give you bad responses, you might want to cut them out of your diet or replace them with others that are better for you.

By using these tips when planning and making meals, you can make balanced meals with sides that help your body heal, improve your health, and make you feel better overall after surgery.

Remember to talk to your doctor or a registered dietitian for personalized dietary advice that is based on your needs and medical condition. With careful planning and mindful choices, you can give your body the nutrients it needs.

CHAPTER 8
SWEET TREATS TO HELP YOU GET BETTER

Indulging in sweet treats while recovering from surgery can be fun and comforting, but it's important to be mindful and limit your intake. Adding sweet treats to your post-surgery diet can help you feel normal and enjoy life during a tough time, but it's important to pick options that help your body heal and stay healthy. In this section, we'll talk about the idea of mindful indulgences for dessert, healthy alternatives, and more.

Desserts to Enjoy With Care

While recovering from surgery, dessert can be a small treat amid pain and dietary restrictions. However, it's important to be aware of how much dessert you eat, taking into account both its nutritional value and how it might affect your recovery.

For example, choosing desserts that are high in nutrients can help your body heal. For example, adding fruits like berries, which are high in antioxidants and vitamins, to desserts can provide bbetter.

Mindfully eating desserts also means watching your portions and taking your time to fully enjoy the flavors. Eating desserts as a treat instead of mindlessly can improve the overall dining experience and make you feel full without overindulging. Also, being aware of how different desserts make you feel after eating them can help you choose the treats that will help your recovery the most.

Healthy Ways to Quench Your Thirst

Traditional desserts like cakes, cookies, and ice cream may be tempting, but many healthy options can satisfy your cravings without setting you back on your recovery.

Experimenting with whole grains, nuts, seeds, and natural sweeteners can help you make tasty desserts that are also good for you.

For example, in baking recipes, switching from refined flour to almond flour or coconut flour can increase the protein and fiber content while still keeping the same number of calories.

Adding healthy foods like avocados, bananas, and Greek yogurt to desserts can also make them creamier and sweeter without using too much sugar or fat. For example, blending frozen bananas with cocoa powder and almond milk makes a chocolate "nice cream" that's both tasty and good for you. Similarly, mixing avocado with cocoa powder and honey makes a chocolate mousse that's rich in healthy fats and antioxidants.

You can add variety to your diet after surgery while still meeting your nutritional needs by trying new desserts. You can do this by using different fruits, alternative sweeteners, or unusual ingredients. There are a lot of ways to make desserts that are both indulgent and healthy.

Having Moderation and Balance When Eating Sweets

Moderation is key to a healthy diet after surgery, even though it's okay to enjoy sweets while you're healing. Eating too many sugary desserts can make inflammation worse, slow down healing, and hurt your overall health, so it's important to find a balance between indulging and moderation when adding sweets to your meals.

One way to practice moderation is to save desserts for special occasions or occasional treats instead of eating them every day. If you think of desserts as a reward for progress or a reason to celebrate, you can enjoy them more mindfully and avoid overindulging. Serving smaller portions or sharing desserts with others can also help you avoid eating too many calories while still satisfying your sweet tooth.

You can lessen the effect of sweet treats on your overall diet by including them in a well-balanced meal plan that also includes lots of fruits, vegetables, lean proteins, and whole grains. Eating nutrient-dense foods along with sweet treats will make sure that your body gets all the nutrients it needs for healing and recovery.

eating sweets while recovering from surgery can make the meal more enjoyable and help you feel better during a tough time. If you eat desserts mindfully, look for healthy alternatives, and do not eat too many, you can enjoy sweets while also supporting your healing and long-term health.

CHAPTER 9

DRINKS THAT CAN HELP YOU HEAL AND STAY HYDRATED

Why staying hydrated after surgery is important:

Maintaining proper hydration is very important for speeding up the healing process and promoting overall recovery after surgery. Hydration is important for many physiological functions, such as tissue repair, circulation, and getting rid of toxins. During surgery, patients often lose fluids, either through blood loss or the body's response to trauma. Anesthesia and pain medications can also make dehydration worse by affecting kidney function.

Making sure you stay hydrated after surgery not only helps your body recover but also makes medications work better and lowers the risk of complications. Drinking enough fluids helps flush out toxins from the body, which is important for preventing infections and promoting optimal wound healing. Staying hydrated can also help with common postoperative symptoms like fatigue, dizziness, and headaches, thereby improving your overall health.

Drinks that are both healthy and tasty:

Choosing the right drinks after surgery can have a big effect on how well you recover by giving you important nutrients while also satisfying your thirst and taste buds. Drinking nutrient-rich drinks not only keeps you hydrated but also helps your body heal by giving it important vitamins, minerals, and antioxidants. Including a variety of drinks in your post-surgery diet keeps things interesting and makes sure you get all the nutrients you need.

These tasty and healthy drinks are good for you after surgery and can help you recover:

1. Herbal Teas: Chamomile, peppermint, and ginger are some examples of herbal teas that can

help people who are recovering from surgery feel better and stay hydrated.

They can also help with nausea, inflammation, and digestive pain which is common after surgery. Herbal teas are also caffeine-free and high in antioxidants, which makes them a great choice for improving overall health and well-being during the recovery period.

2. Homemade broths and soups: Broths and soups made from scratch with nutrient-dense foods like bone broth, vegetables, and lean proteins can keep the body hydrated and provide essential nutrients. These liquid-based meals are easy to digest and can be changed to fit dietary needs and preferences.

 The warmth of soups and broths can also provide comfort and relief, especially in the early stages of recovery when the appetite may be weak.

3. Fruit and Vegetable Juices: Freshly squeezed fruit and vegetable juices are full of antioxidants,

vitamins, and minerals, which makes them a great choice for boosting your immune system and helping you heal after surgery. Using a variety of fruits and vegetables in your juices ensures that you get a wide range of nutrients, like vitamin C, potassium, and folate, which are important for healing and tissue repair. However, it's important to choose juices that you make yourself or that don't contain added sugar.

4. Protein Shakes and Smoothies: Protein shakes and smoothies are easy to make and are great for people who have recently had surgery or who need extra protein to help their wounds heal and tissues grow back. By mixing protein sources like whey, plant-based protein powders, or Greek yogurt with fruits, vegetables, and healthy fats, you can make a nutrient-dense drink that helps your muscles recover and your overall nutrition.

How to Make Healing Infusions and Tonics:

Adding healing tonics and infusions to your diet after surgery can help with healing even more while keeping you hydrated and boosting your nutrition. These mixtures often contain medicinal herbs, spices, and other natural ingredients that are known to be healing, which makes them a great addition to regular medical treatment. Making your healing tonics and infusions lets you tailor them to your personal tastes and health concerns.

Some ideas for tonics and infusions that can help you feel better:

1. Turmeric Golden Milk: Golden milk, sometimes called turmeric latte, is a traditional Ayurvedic drink that is known for helping the immune system and reducing inflammation. To make it, heat milk (dairy or plant-based) with ground turmeric, ginger, cinnamon, and a little black pepper to help the turmeric dissolve. Add honey or maple syrup to taste and drink before bed as a soothing and healing drink.

2. Lemon Ginger Detox Infusion: Fresh lemon slices, ginger root, and mint leaves steeped in hot water make this a refreshing and detoxifying drink. Lemon is high in vitamin C and antioxidants, and ginger helps digestion and reduces inflammation. Drink this energizing infusion throughout the day to stay hydrated and help your body detox after surgery.

Hibiscus Rosehip Tea: A blend of hibiscus and rosehip flowers makes a tart and floral drink that is full of vitamin C and antioxidants. It is a great choice for supporting immune health and collagen production while you are recovering. To make this tea, steep dried hibiscus flowers, and rosehip berries in hot water for a colorful and flavorful drink that you can enjoy hot or cold.

Peppermint Lavender Relaxation Tonic: This soothing tonic is made from fresh peppermint leaves, dried lavender flowers, and a hint of honey. It is a fragrant and relaxing drink that is great for easing stress and promoting relaxation after surgery. Steep the peppermint and lavender in hot water for a few minutes, strain, and add honey to taste.

Sip this calming tonic before bed or during moments of rest to ease tension and encourage restful sleep.

Finally, drinking nourishing and hydrating drinks after surgery is important for helping the body heal and speeding up the recovery process as a whole. Nutrient-dense drinks like herbal teas, homemade broths, fresh juices, and healing tonics can help people get the most nutrients while staying hydrated and comfortable during the recovery period. Trying out different recipes and flavors adds variety and interest to the recovery process.

CHAPTER 10
HOW TO PLAN MEALS AND COOK IN BIG GRIPS

Meal planning and batch cooking are important parts of a successful post-surgery diet plan.

These methods not only make preparing meals easier, but they also make sure that people who are recovering from surgery can get healthy meals without too much stress or work. By carefully planning meals and using batch cooking methods, people can speed up their recovery and improve their health in the long term.

Making meal prep easier for recovery

Getting ready for meals and staying healthy can be hard in the days and weeks after surgery because people are often physically and emotionally tired. But, good nutrition is important for helping the body heal and avoiding complications, so it's important to focus on efficiency and convenience when planning meals during this time.

• Making easy, healthy meals that don't take a lot of work or time to cook.

• Buying tools and gadgets for the kitchen that make cooking easier, like an instant pot or soup pot.

• Stocking up on basic foods that are easy to use in many different recipes, like lean proteins, whole grains, and lots of fruits and veggies.

1. Ask family or friends to help you plan meals, either by cooking meals ahead of time or by going food shopping and preparing the ingredients.

• Using pre-packaged or convenience foods less often and making meals at home with healthy items more often when they can.

By making dinner prep easier and focusing on efficiency, people can make sure they have access to healthy meals while they're recovering without adding extra stress or burden.

How to Cook a Lot of Meals at Once and Freeze Them

Batch cooking is a great way to make meal preparation easier and make sure that people always have access to healthy meals, even when they're not feeling very energetic. By setting aside a few hours a week to make big batches of meals that can be divided up and stored for later use, people can greatly reduce the time and effort needed to cook every day.

Some ideas that work well for making a lot of food at once are soups, stews, casseroles, and grain-based dishes.

Spending money on good storage containers that can go in the fridge and keep food fresh for a long time.

• Writing the date and contents of containers on them to make sure they are rotated properly and keep food from going to waste.

• Using a range of tastes and products to keep meals interesting and filling.

• Trying out different ways to cook, like baking, sautéing, and braising, to make batch-cooked meals more interesting.

• Making plans ahead of time to set aside time each week for batch cooking to stay organized and on track.

By using these tips, people can effectively use batch cooking to keep a steady supply of healthy meals while they are recovering. This will save them time from having to cook every day and make sure they have access to healthy food when they need it most.

How to Make Successful Meal Plans

Planning meals is an important part of a healthy diet after surgery because it gives people structure and direction as they go through their recovery.

A good meal plan takes into account each person's dietary needs, preferences, and restrictions, as well as includes a balance of nutrients to help with healing and overall health.

When making a meal plan for recovery after surgery, think about the following things:

• Discuss your nutritional needs and any special dietary restrictions or suggestions with a medical professional or registered dietitian.

To help the body heal and get the nutrients it needs, eat a wide range of nutrient-dense foods, such as lean proteins, whole grains, healthy fats, and lots of fruits and veggies.

• Planning meals and snacks to eat at regular times throughout the day to keep your energy level steady and help your body absorb nutrients better.

• Changing portion sizes and how often you eat depending on your appetite, level of activity, and progress in recovery.

• The ability to adapt to changes in taste, hunger, or dietary needs while the person is recovering.

• Using meal prep and batch cooking to make the process of making meals easier and make sure that healthy meals are always available.

Individuals can improve their post-surgery recovery and long-term health and wellness by carefully creating a personalized meal plan that takes into account their specific needs and preferences. Seeking advice from medical professionals or registered dietitians can also be very helpful in creating an effective and long-lasting meal plan for recovery.

CHAPTER 11

DEALING WITH DIETARY PROBLEMS AND LIMITATIONS

Maintaining a well-balanced diet is very important for a quick recovery and long-term health.

This means dealing with common dietary restrictions, changing recipes to fit specific needs, and handling problems with ease. Knowing these ideas helps patients better control their nutritional intake after surgery, which speeds up recovery and improves overall health.

Taking Care of Common Dietary Limitations After Surgery

People often have to follow certain dietary restrictions after surgery, depending on their procedure and health condition. These restrictions usually include not being able to eat certain food groups, like high-fat, high-sugar, or high-fiber foods, and not being able to drink alcohol or caffeine. These restrictions are put in place to avoid complications, help with healing, and support the body's recovery process. For example, after the gastrointestinal surge,

Making Changes to Recipes to Fit Needs

It takes creativity and knowledge of nutritional needs and restrictions to change recipes to fit specific dietary needs after surgery. This can mean swapping ingredients, changing the way food is cooked, or changing portion sizes to make sure that dietary guidelines are followed. For example, people with diabetes may need to replace sugar in recipes with other sweeteners, and people with lactose intolerance may choose dairy-free alternatives.

Some easy ways to deal with diet problems

Navigating dietary challenges post-surgery can be daunting, but with careful planning and support, individuals can overcome these obstacles with ease. One essential tip is to plan meals and snacks, ensuring they align with dietary recommendations and meet nutritional needs. This involves creating meal plans that include a variety of nutrient-rich foods while considering portion sizes and frequency of meals to support healing and prevent overeating. Additionally, experimenting with new recipes and cooking methods can help keep meals interesting and enjoyable, reducing the temptation to stray from dietary restrictions.

It's also crucial to communicate openly with healthcare providers and seek support from family and friends to maintain motivation and accountability throughout the recovery process. Finally, practicing mindful eating techniques, such as paying attention to hunger and fullness cues, can help prevent overeating and promote a healthy relationship with food post-surgery.

By implementing these tips and strategies, individuals can navigate dietary challenges with confidence and support their long-term wellness goals.

A complete guide to the best diet after surgery for people who have just been diagnosed, with healing recipes, meal plans, and expert advice for long-term health.

An optimal post-surgery diet is important for helping the body heal and promoting long-term health after surgery. This complete guide gives helpful information on how to make a nourishing post-surgery diet, including healing recipes, customisable meal plans, and expert tips for staying healthy.

Understanding Why a Diet After Surgery Is Important

A post-surgery diet is very important for helping the body heal, avoiding complications, and maintaining overall health. It gives the body the nutrients it needs for energy production, tissue repair, and immune function, which makes sure the recovery process goes smoothly.

A well-balanced diet can also help control inflammation, lower the risk of infection, and support optimal wound healing, which speeds up the return to normal activities.

Recipes that will help you heal after surgery

Adding healing recipes to your diet after surgery can help you get more nutrients and speed up the healing process. These recipes are made to be easy to digest, nutrient-rich, and full of important vitamins, minerals, and antioxidants.

Homemade soups, broths, smoothies, and purees are all examples of healing foods that can help you stay hydrated, get important nutrients, and feel better while you're recovering.

Meal plans that can be changed to fit each person's needs

To stick to a post-surgery diet, it's important to make meal plans that are flexible and based on each person's dietary needs and preferences.

These plans should include a variety of nutrient-rich foods from all food groups, like fruits, vegetables, whole grains, lean proteins, and healthy fats. Meal timing and portion control should also be thought about to keep people from overeating and help digestion.

Tips from experts for long-term health

In addition to following a post-surgery diet, following expert tips for long-term wellness can also improve your health and well-being. For example, these tips might include staying hydrated by drinking lots of water throughout the day, doing regular physical activity to improve circulation and healing, and getting enough sleep to help your immune system work and repair tissues.

Adopting the best post-surgery diet is important for speeding up recovery, avoiding complications, and maintaining long-term health. By learning about the importance of a post-surgery diet and incorporating healing recipes, customisable meal plans, and expert tips into their daily routine, people can improve their nutrition and support a faster recovery. With careful planning, support, and guidance from healthcare professionals, people can navigate

CHAPTER 12
BEYOND THE PLATE: HOLISTIC APPROACHES TO HEALING

It's impossible to overstate how important holistic approaches are for healing and recovery.

Medical interventions are very important, but addressing the mind-body connection is becoming more and more seen as key to the best results.

The holistic approach recognizes that healing is more than just physical symptoms; it includes mental, emotional, and even spiritual aspects.

By looking into how these aspects are connected, people can unwind and feel better.

Mind-Body Connection Is Important for Recovery

The mind-body connection is the complex relationship between mental and physical health. It recognizes that our thoughts, feelings, and beliefs can have a big effect on our physical health and vice versa. When it comes to recovery, fostering a positive mind-body connection can make healing much more effective. Studies have shown that people who keep a positive attitude and do practices like meditation, mindfulness, and visualizing

Stress hormones are controlled by the mind-body connection, which can help with recovery. Long-term stress has been linked to many health problems, such as slower wound healing, more inflammation, and weaker immune systems.

People can lower their stress levels and improve their health by using relaxation techniques like deep breathing, progressive muscle relaxation, and guided imagery in their daily lives.

In addition, the mind-body connection is very important for managing pain. How much pain someone feels isn't just based on how badly their tissues are damaged; it's also affected by emotions like fear, anxiety, and depression.

By dealing with these emotions through cognitive-behavioral therapy (CBT) and biofeedback, people can effectively lower how much pain they feel and improve their overall quality of life during treatment.

Using relaxation techniques as part of daily life

It is important to include relaxation techniques in your daily life if you want to heal and be healthy. These techniques work to counteract the negative effects of stress on the body and mind, creating a state of calmness and balance that is good for recovery. Mindfulness meditation is one of the best relaxation techniques for promoting relaxation and lowering stress levels.

Focusing on the present moment without judging it is what mindfulness meditation is all about. It helps people develop inner peace and awareness. Regular practice of mindfulness meditation has been shown to significantly lower stress, anxiety, and depression, as well as improve sleep quality and overall mental health. By setting aside just a few minutes each day to do mindfulness meditation, individuals can

Besides mindfulness meditation, you can also use progressive muscle relaxation, deep breathing exercises, and guided imagery as part of your daily routine to help you relax and lower your stress. Progressive muscle relaxation involves slowly tensing and relaxing different muscle groups in the body, which helps release physical tension and promote a sense of relaxation. Deep breathing exercises, such as diaphragmatic breathing,

Creating a Healing Community to Help Each Other

Making a supportive community is important for healing and recovery. Social support helps people deal with the challenges of illness and injury by giving them emotional support, practical help, and a sense of belonging.

Having a strong support network, whether it's family, friends, support groups, or healthcare professionals, can make a person much more resilient and better able to get through the recovery process.

One of the best things about social support is that it can help people who are recovering from feeling lonely and alone. By surrounding themselves with caring, understanding, and affirming people who understand and validate their experiences, people can feel more connected and supported, which lowers their risk of developing depression and anxiety. Social support can also help with daily tasks like transportation and meal prep.

A supportive community can offer more than just emotional and practical support. It can also provide useful resources and information to help with the recovery process. Support groups, whether they're in person or online, give people a chance to talk about their problems, learn from others, and get access to useful resources and information. Healthcare professionals like doctors, nurses, therapists, and counselors can also be very helpful by giving advice, support, and encouragement.

Additionally, creating a supportive community includes more than just close family and friends. Volunteering with community groups, religious institutions, and community organizations can provide extra sources of support and connection, creating a sense of belonging and purpose.

People who are recovering can improve their lives by actively seeking out and nurturing supportive relationships in their community.

For that reason, holistic approaches to healing are more than just medical interventions; they look at how the mind, body, and spirit are all connected to promote overall health. Recognizing the importance of the mind-body connection, incorporating relaxation techniques into daily routines, and creating a supportive community can help people become more resilient and speed up their recovery.

CONCLUSION

This book, "The Peacemaker Surgery Dietary Cookbook," has helped me understand and follow the best post-surgery diet. It has been a complete guide to long-term health and healing, from learning about Peacemaker Surgery to exploring the science behind the dietary needs for recovery, each chapter has given me useful information on how to nourish the body and speed up the healing process.

Preparing the kitchen for success is very important, as shown in Chapter 3, which talks about necessary tools, stocking the pantry, and meal planning. Chapters 4–9 talked about the healing power of whole foods, including tasty soups, filling main dishes, refreshing sides, and healthy sweet treats, stressing the importance of balanced nutrition in every meal.

Additionally, Chapter 10 talked about practical ways to plan meals and cook in bulk, which will make following dietary requirements easier and more convenient in the long run. Chapter 11 talked about common dietary problems and restrictions and advised on how to adapt and get around them. Finally, Chapter 12 took the focus off of the plate and pushed for healing methods that include the mind-body connection and community support.

This cookbook is more than just a collection of recipes; it's a road map to optimal recovery and long-term wellness. It includes not only healing recipes and meal plans but also expert advice and a holistic view. By following the principles outlined in this guide, people going through Peacemaker Surgery can start a journey towards complete healing, supported by healthy food, mindful practices, and a supportive community.